WEEK CYCLE 1	MONDAY	TUESDAY	WEDNESDAY	THURSDAY	FRIDAY

WEEK CYCLE 2	MONDAY	TUESDAY	WEDNESDAY	THURSDAY	FRIDAY

WEEK CYCLE 3	MONDAY	TUESDAY	WEDNESDAY	THURSDAY	FRIDAY

WEEK CYCLE4	MONDAY	TUESDAY	WEDNESDAY	THURSDAY	FRIDAY

MEDICAL INFORMATION

WEEK CYCLE 5	MONDAY	TUESDAY	WEDNESDAY	THURSDAY	FRIDAY

WEEK CYCLE 6	MONDAY	TUESDAY	WEDNESDAY	THURSDAY	FRIDAY

WEEK CYCLE 7	MONDAY	TUESDAY	WEDNESDAY	THURSDAY	FRIDAY

WEEK CYCLE 8	MONDAY	TUESDAY	WEDNESDAY	THURSDAY	FRIDAY

MEDICAL INFORMATION

OTHER DATES TO REMEMBER

OTHER DATES TO REMEMBER

MEDICAL INFORMATION

OTHER DATES TO REMEMBER

OTHER DATES TO REMEMBER

MEDICAL INFORMATION

OTHER DATES TO REMEMBER

OTHER DATES TO REMEMBER

MEDICAL INFORMATION

OTHER DATES TO REMEMBER

OTHER DATES TO REMEMBER

MEDICAL INFORMATION

NAME (DOCTOR/NURSE/SUPPORT GROUP)	TELEPHONE NUMBER	CLINIC LOCATION

MEDICAL INFORMATION

NAME (DOCTOR/NURSE/SUPPORT GROUP)	TELEPHONE NUMBER	CLINIC LOCATION

MEDICAL INFORMATION

USEFUL CONTACTS

NAME	TELEPHONE NUMBER	ADDRESS

MEDICAL INFORMATION

USEFUL CONTACTS

NAME	TELEPHONE NUMBER	ADDRESS

MEDICAL INFORMATION

TREATMENT MEDICATION PRESCRIBED

TREATMENT/MEDICATION	DOCTOR PRESCRIBED BY	DATE

MEDICAL INFORMATION

TREATMENT MEDICATION PRESCRIBED

TREATMENT/MEDICATION	DOCTOR PRESCRIBED BY	DATE

MEDICAL INFORMATION

CYCLE 1	DAY	DATE	BLOOD COUNT LOW/HIGH	MOOD, SIDE EFFECTS & COMMENTS	SOLUTION	Sugar level mmol	Temp C
Example: CYCLE 1	Example: DAY 1	Example: 1st January 2018	Example: blood count drops or rises.	Example: nausea/vomiting, dizzy, fatigue, rash, pain, breathless, loss of appetite, constipation, diarrhoea, fever, loss of hair, sore / dry mouth, depressed or duration of treatment and type.	Example: a sip of water, rest, eat.	Example: 5.4	Example: 36.7
CYCLE 1	DAY 1						
	DAY 2						
	DAY 3						
	DAY 4						
	DAY 5						
	DAY 6						
	DAY 7						
	DAY 8						
	DAY 9						
	DAY 10						
	DAY 11						
	DAY 12						
	DAY 13						
	DAY 14						
	DAY 15						
	DAY 16						
	DAY 17						
	DAY 18						
	DAY 19						
	DAY 20						
	DAY 21						

CYCLE 2	DAY	DATE	BLOOD COUNT LOW/HIGH	MOOD, SIDE EFFECTS & COMMENTS	SOLUTION	Sugar level mmol	Temp C
Example: CYCLE 2	*Example: DAY 1*	*Example: 1st January 2018*	*Example: blood count drops or rises.*	*Example: nausea/vomiting, dizzy, fatigue, rash, pain, breathless, loss of appetite, constipation, diarrhoea, fever, loss of hair, sore / dry mouth, depressed or duration of treatment and type.*	*Example: a sip of water, rest, eat.*	*Example: 5.4*	*Example: 36.7*
CYCLE 2	DAY 1						
	DAY 2						
	DAY 3						
	DAY 4						
	DAY 5						
	DAY 6						
	DAY 7						
	DAY 8						
	DAY 9						
	DAY 10						
	DAY 11						
	DAY 12						
	DAY 13						
	DAY 14						
	DAY 15						
	DAY 16						
	DAY 17						
	DAY 18						
	DAY 19						
	DAY 20						
	DAY 21						

CYCLE 3	DAY	DATE	BLOOD COUNT LOW/HIGH	MOOD, SIDE EFFECTS & COMMENTS	SOLUTION	Sugar level mmol	Temp C
Example: CYCLE 3	Example: DAY 1	Example: 1st January 2018	Example: blood count drops or rises.	Example: nausea/vomiting, dizzy, fatigue, rash, pain, breathless, loss of appetite, constipation, diarrhoea, fever, loss of hair, sore / dry mouth, depressed or duration of treatment and type.	Example: a sip of water, rest, eat.	Example: 5.4	Example: 36.7
CYCLE 3	DAY 1						
	DAY 2						
	DAY 3						
	DAY 4						
	DAY 5						
	DAY 6						
	DAY 7						
	DAY 8						
	DAY 9						
	DAY 10						
	DAY 11						
	DAY 12						
	DAY 13						
	DAY 14						
	DAY 15						
	DAY 16						
	DAY 17						
	DAY 18						
	DAY 19						
	DAY 20						
	DAY 21						

CYCLE 4	DAY	DATE	BLOOD COUNT LOW/HIGH	MOOD, SIDE EFFECTS & COMMENTS	SOLUTION	Sugar level mmol	Temp C
Example: CYCLE 4	Example: DAY 1	Example: 1st January 2018	Example: blood count drops or rises.	Example: nausea/vomiting, dizzy, fatigue, rash, pain, breathless, loss of appetite, constipation, diarrhoea, fever, loss of hair, sore / dry mouth, depressed or duration of treatment and type.	Example: a sip of water, rest, eat.	Example: 5.4	Example: 36.7
CYCLE 4	DAY 1						
	DAY 2						
	DAY 3						
	DAY 4						
	DAY 5						
	DAY 6						
	DAY 7						
	DAY 8						
	DAY 9						
	DAY 10						
	DAY 11						
	DAY 12						
	DAY 13						
	DAY 14						
	DAY 15						
	DAY 16						
	DAY 17						
	DAY 18						
	DAY 19						
	DAY 20						
	DAY 21						

CYCLE 5	DATE	BLOOD COUNT LOW/HIGH	MOOD, SIDE EFFECTS & COMMENTS	SOLUTION	Sugar level mmol	Temp C
Example: CYCLE 5	Example: 1st January 2018	Example: blood count drops or rises.	Example: nausea/vomiting, dizzy, fatigue, rash, pain, breathless, loss of appetite, constipation, diarrhoea, fever, loss of hair, sore / dry mouth, depressed or duration of treatment and type.	Example: a sip of water, rest, eat.	Example: 5.4	Example: 36.7
Example: DAY 1						
CYCLE 5 DAY 1						
DAY 2						
DAY 3						
DAY 4						
DAY 5						
DAY 6						
DAY 7						
DAY 8						
DAY 9						
DAY 10						
DAY 11						
DAY 12						
DAY 13						
DAY 14						
DAY 15						
DAY 16						
DAY 17						
DAY 18						
DAY 19						
DAY 20						
DAY 21						

CYCLE 6	DATE	BLOOD COUNT LOW/HIGH	MOOD, SIDE EFFECTS & COMMENTS	SOLUTION	Sugar level mmol	Temp C
Example: CYCLE 6	Example: 1st January 2018	Example: blood count drops or rises.	Example: nausea/vomiting, dizzy, fatigue, rash, pain, breathless, loss of appetite, constipation, diarrhoea, fever, loss of hair, sore / dry moutth, depressed or duration of treatment and type.	Example: a sip of water, rest, eat.	Example: 5.4	Example: 36.7
CYCLE 6						
DAY 1						
DAY 2						
DAY 3						
DAY 4						
DAY 5						
DAY 6						
DAY 7						
DAY 8						
DAY 9						
DAY 10						
DAY 11						
DAY 12						
DAY 13						
DAY 14						
DAY 15						
DAY 16						
DAY 17						
DAY 18						
DAY 19						
DAY 20						
DAY 21						

CYCLE 7		DATE	BLOOD COUNT LOW/HIGH	MOOD, SIDE EFFECTS & COMMENTS	SOLUTION	Sugar level mmol	Temp C
Example: CYCLE 7	Example: DAY 1	Example: 1st January 2018	Example: blood count drops or rises.	Example: nausea/vomiting, dizzy, fatigue, rash, pain, breathless, loss of appetite, constipation, diarrhoea, fever, loss of hair, sore / dry mouth, depressed or duration of treatment and type.	Example: a sip of water, rest, eat.	Example: 5.4	Example: 36.7
CYCLE 7	DAY 1						
	DAY 2						
	DAY 3						
	DAY 4						
	DAY 5						
	DAY 6						
	DAY 7						
	DAY 8						
	DAY 9						
	DAY 10						
	DAY 11						
	DAY 12						
	DAY 13						
	DAY 14						
	DAY 15						
	DAY 16						
	DAY 17						
	DAY 18						
	DAY 19						
	DAY 20						
	DAY 21						

CYCLE 8		DATE	BLOOD COUNT LOW/HIGH	MOOD, SIDE EFFECTS & COMMENTS	SOLUTION	Sugar level mmol	Temp C
Example: CYCLE 8	Example: DAY 1	Example: 1st January 2018	Example: blood count drops or rises.	Example: nausea/vomiting, dizzy, fatigue, rash, pain, breathless, loss of appetite, constipation, diarrhoea, fever, loss of hair, sore / dry mouth, depressed or duration of treatment and type.	Example: a sip of water, rest, eat.	Example: 5.4	Example: 36.7
CYCLE 8	DAY 1						
	DAY 2						
	DAY 3						
	DAY 4						
	DAY 5						
	DAY 6						
	DAY 7						
	DAY 8						
	DAY 9						
	DAY 10						
	DAY 11						
	DAY 12						
	DAY 13						
	DAY 14						
	DAY 15						
	DAY 16						
	DAY 17						
	DAY 18						
	DAY 19						
	DAY 20						
	DAY 21						

FURTHER NOTES

Feelings, thoughts & doodles

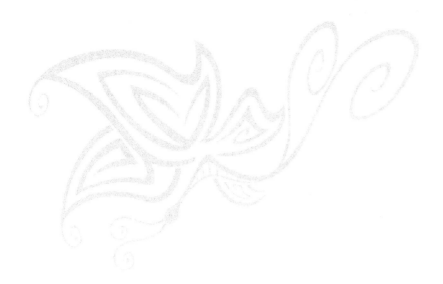

Know yourself.

FURTHER NOTES

Thoughts & doodles

The point of power is always in the present moment.

FURTHER NOTES

Thoughts & doodles

Love is all that matters in
this world.

FURTHER NOTES

Thoughts & doodles

Look within to find your treasures.

FURTHER NOTES

Thoughts & doodles

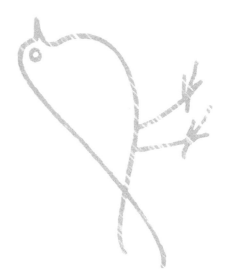

Accept and acknowledge your feelings whether positive or negative.

FURTHER NOTES

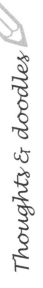

Thoughts & doodles

Rely on Divine guidance and wisdom to protect you at all times.

FURTHER NOTES

Thoughts & doodles

Create peacefulness in your mind and trust your inner wisdom.

FURTHER NOTES

Thoughts & doodles

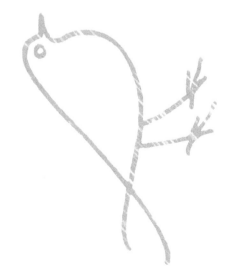

Believe in yourself at all times.

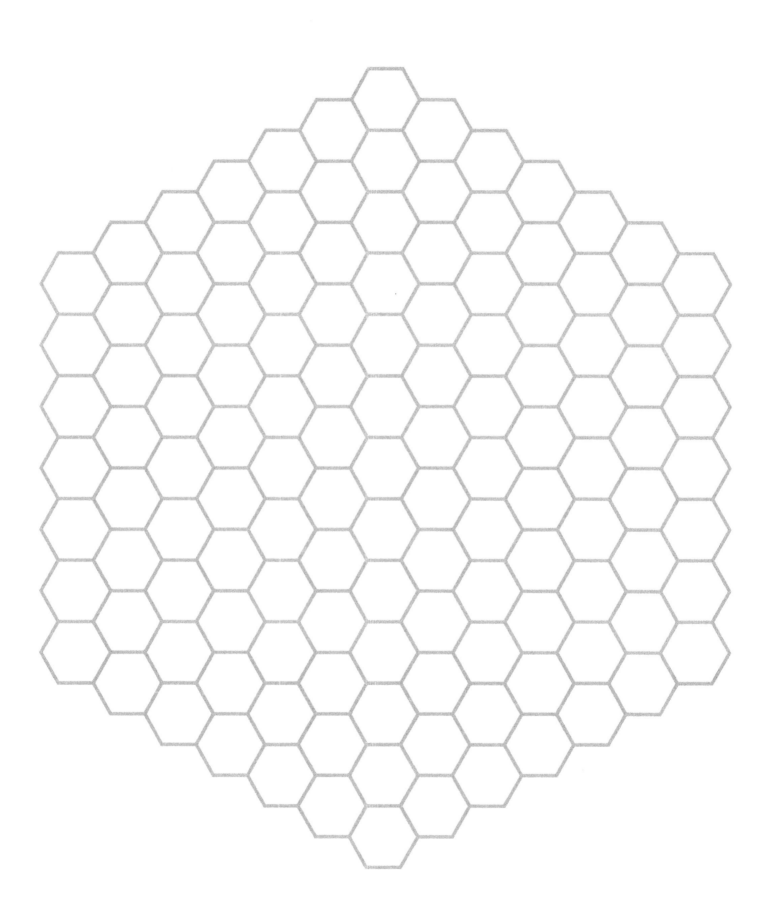

NOTES

NOTES

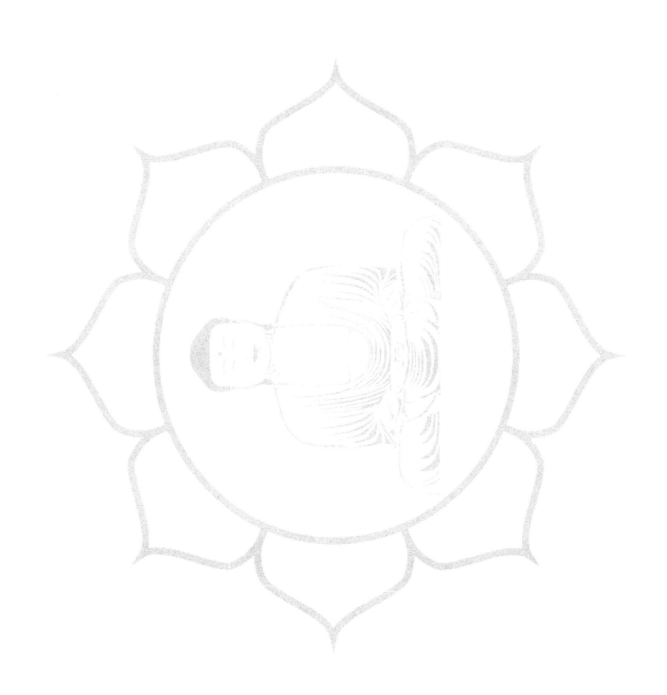

NOTES

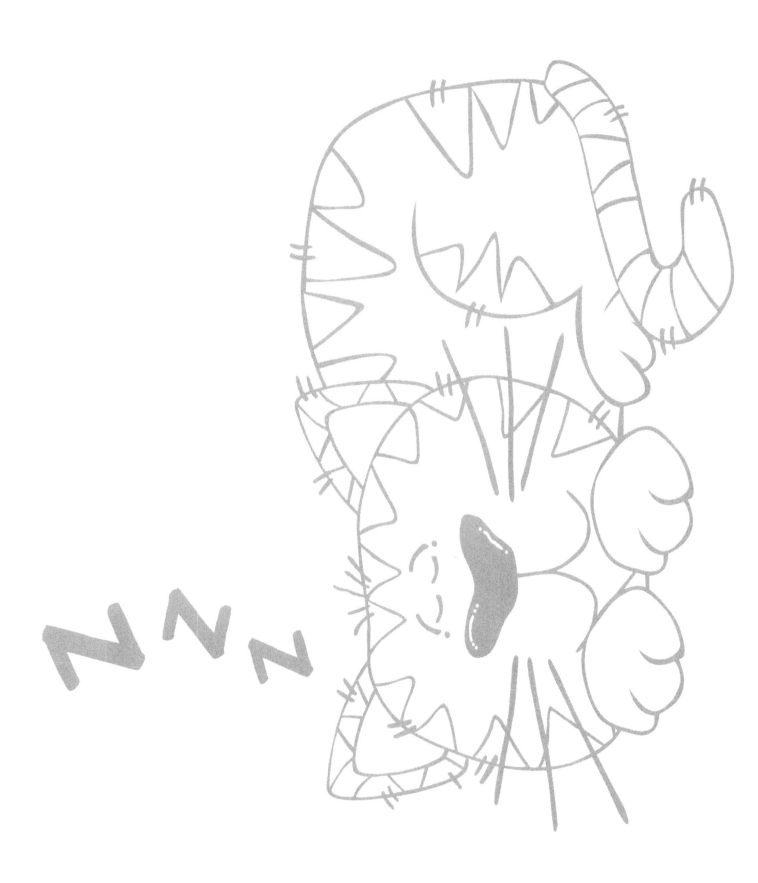

NOTES

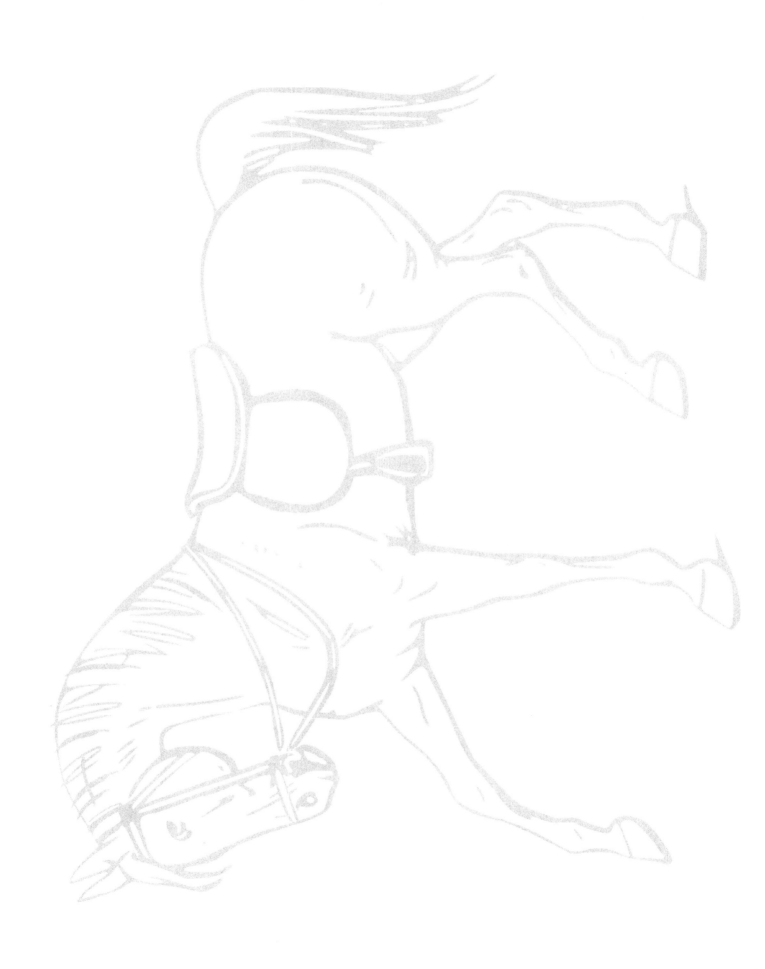

NOTES

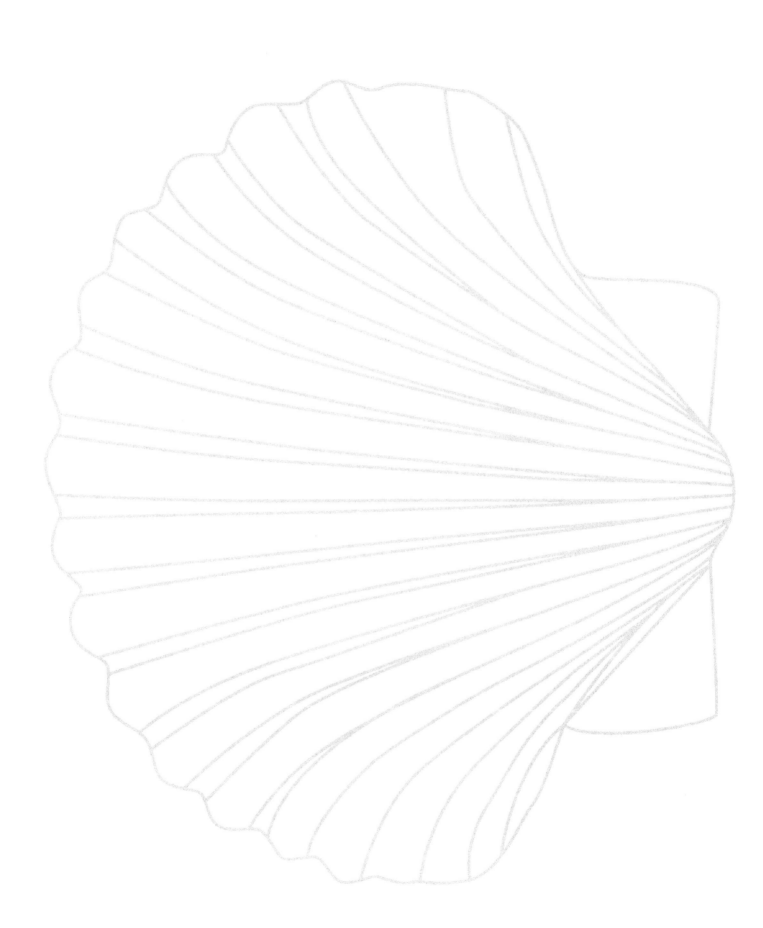

NOTES

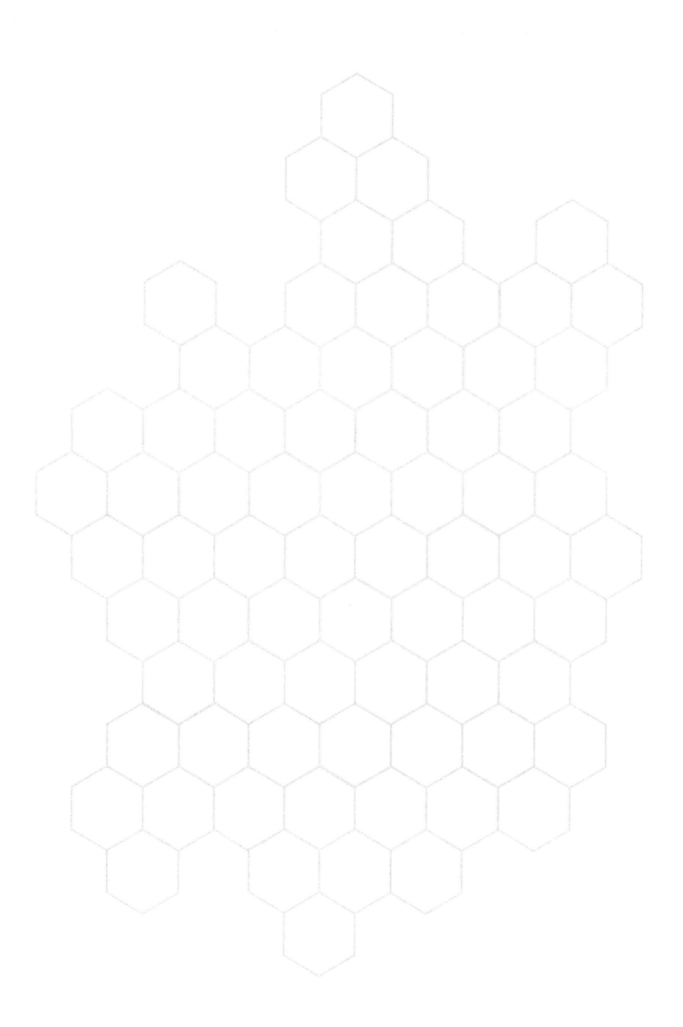

NOTES

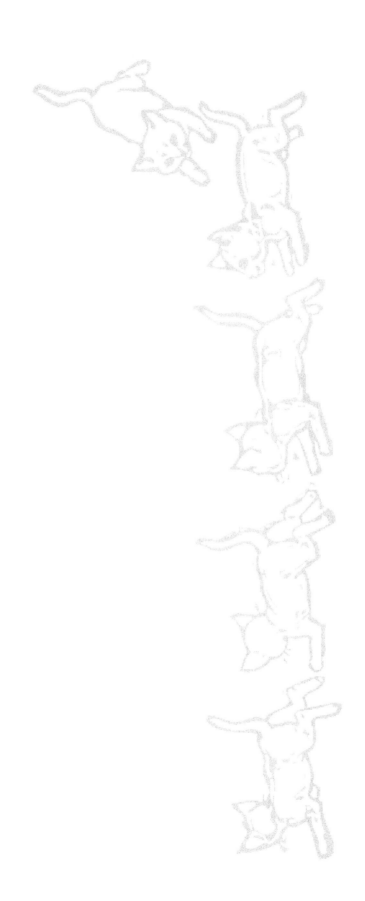

NOTES

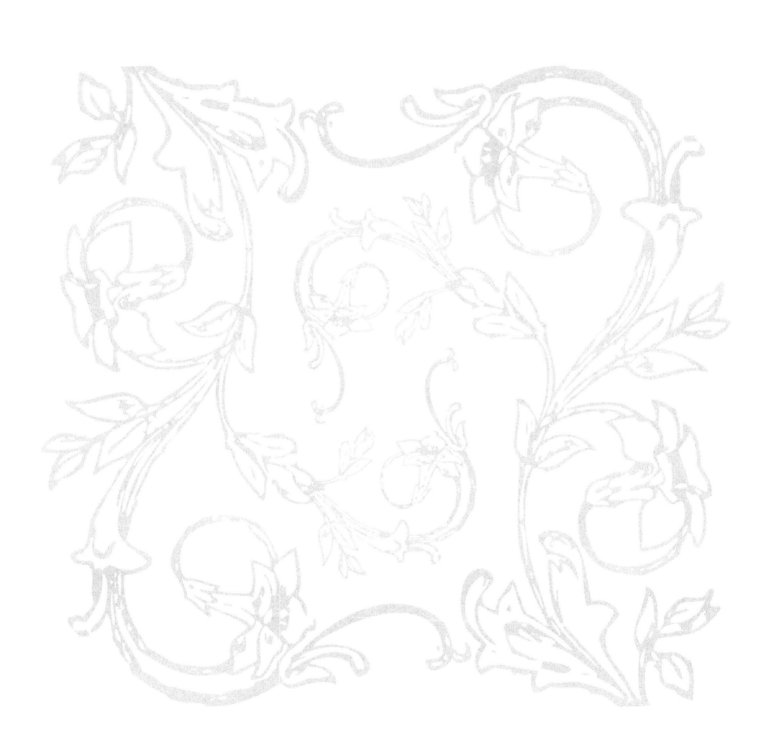

NOTES

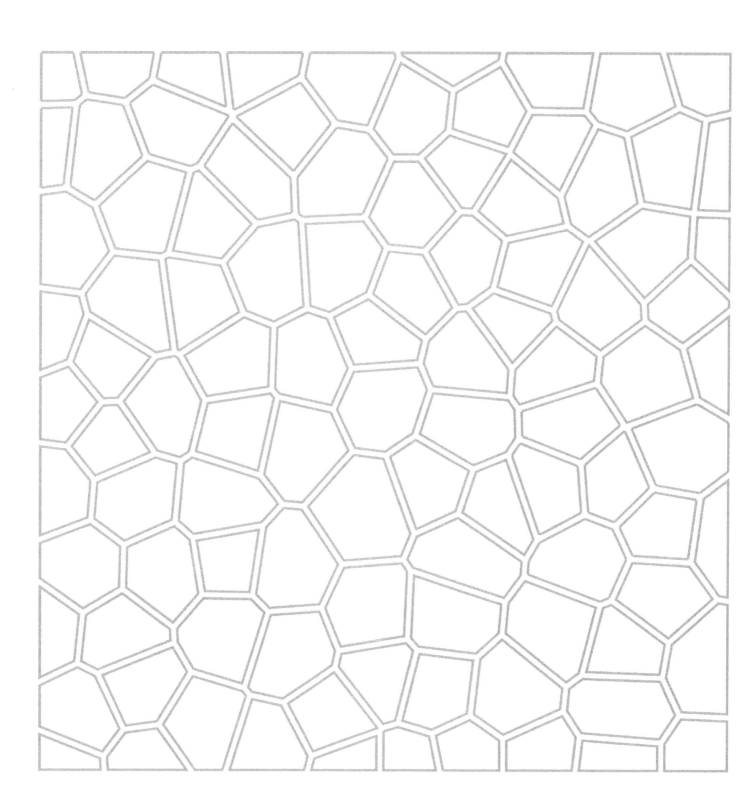

NOTES

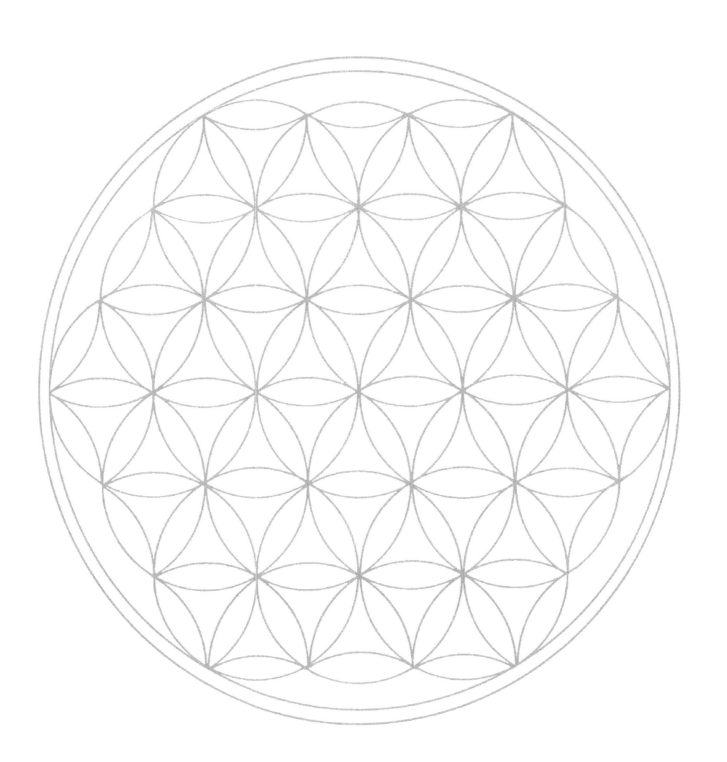

NOTES

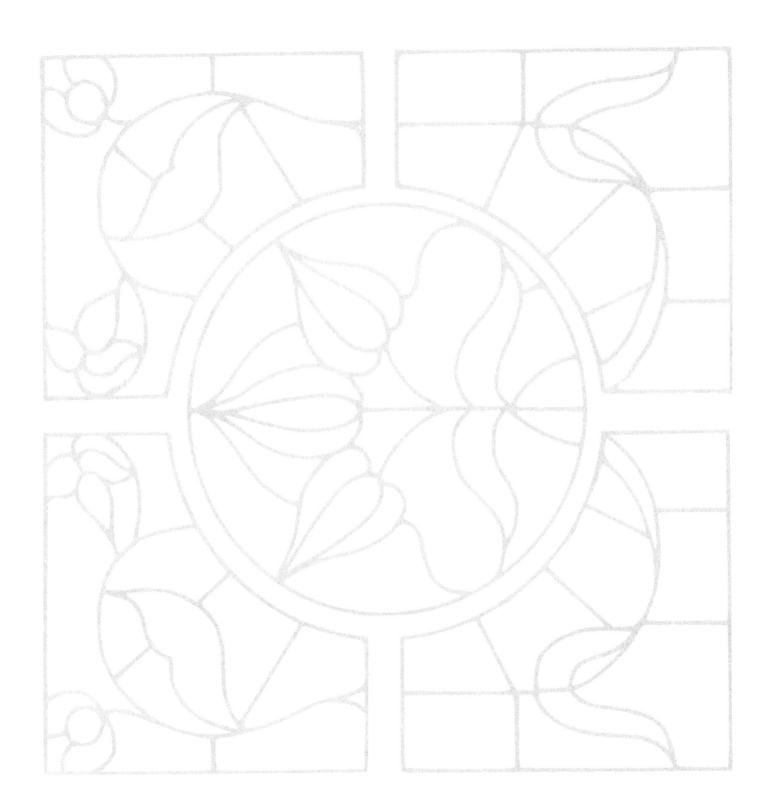

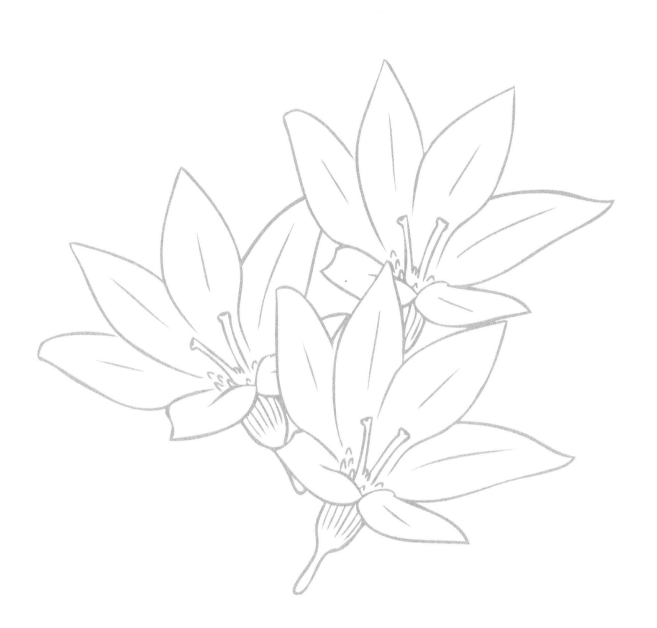

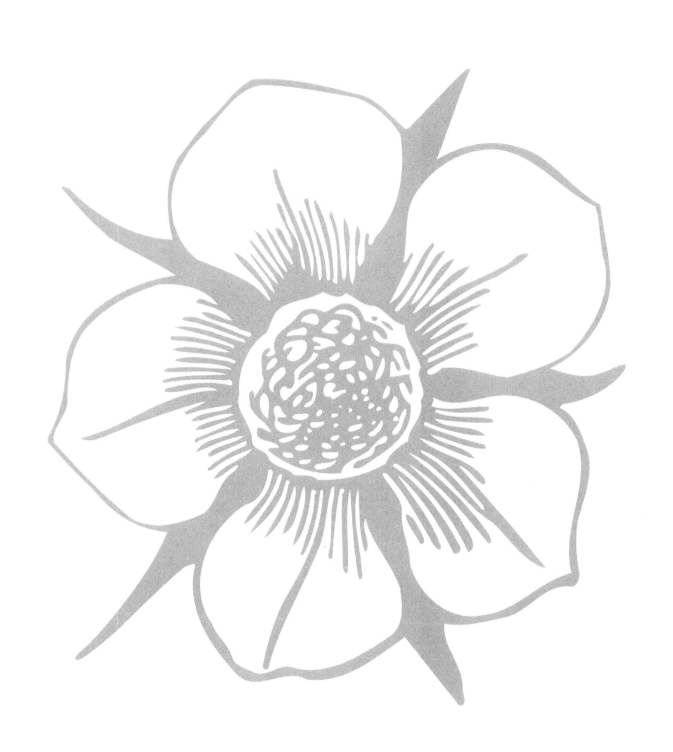

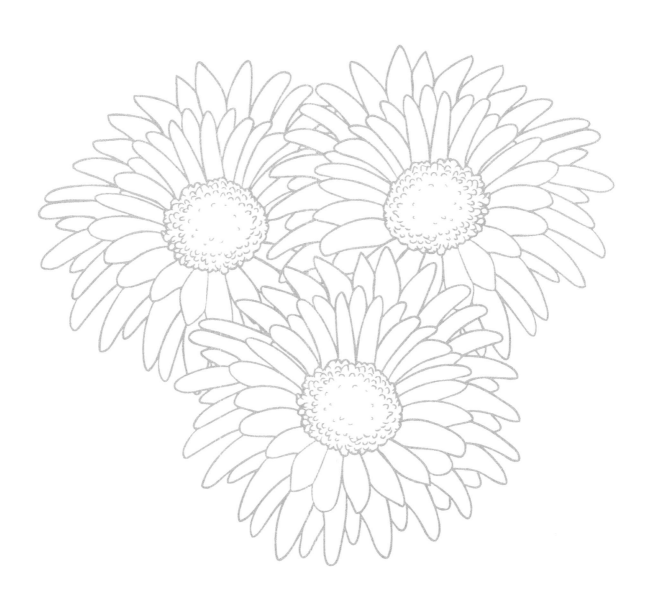

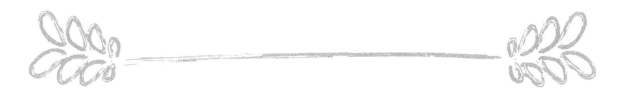

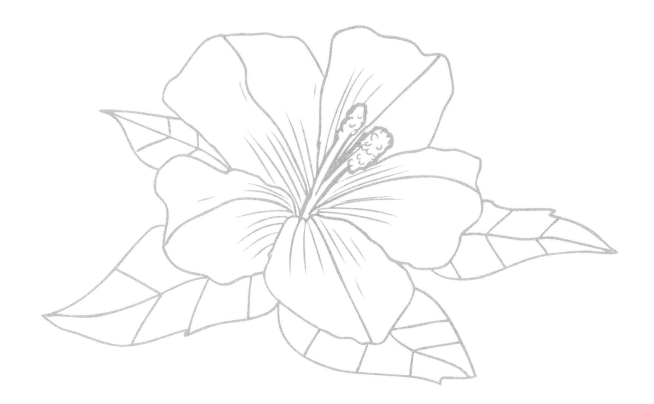

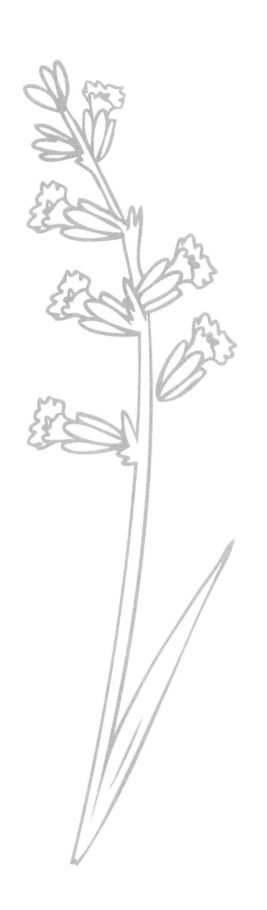

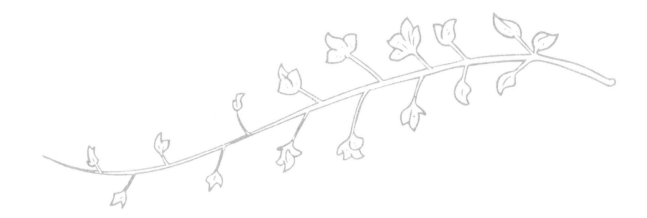

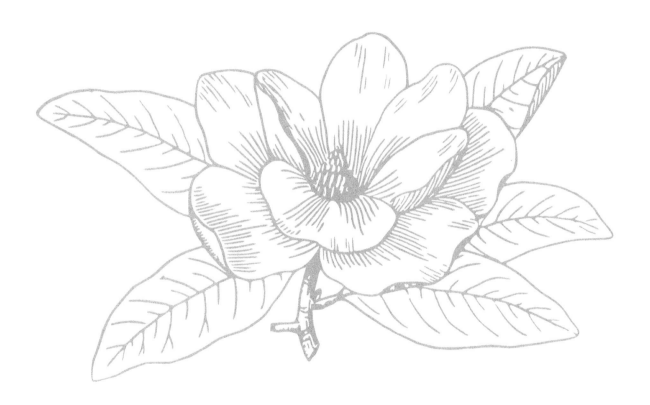

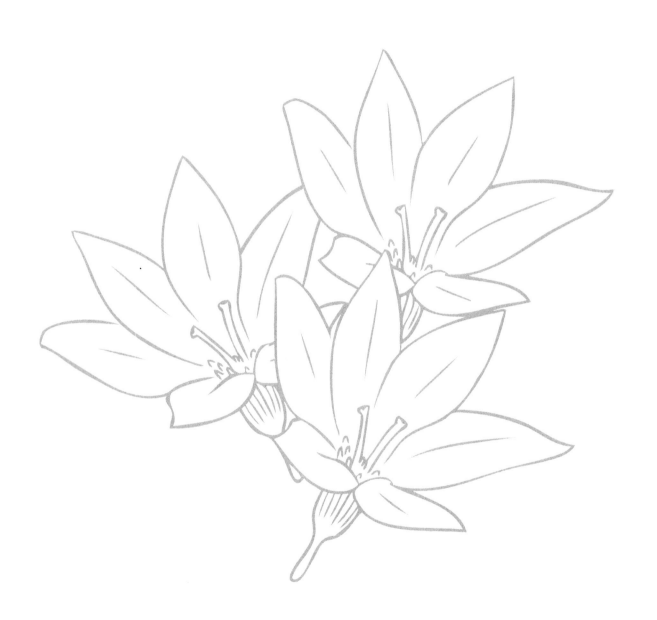

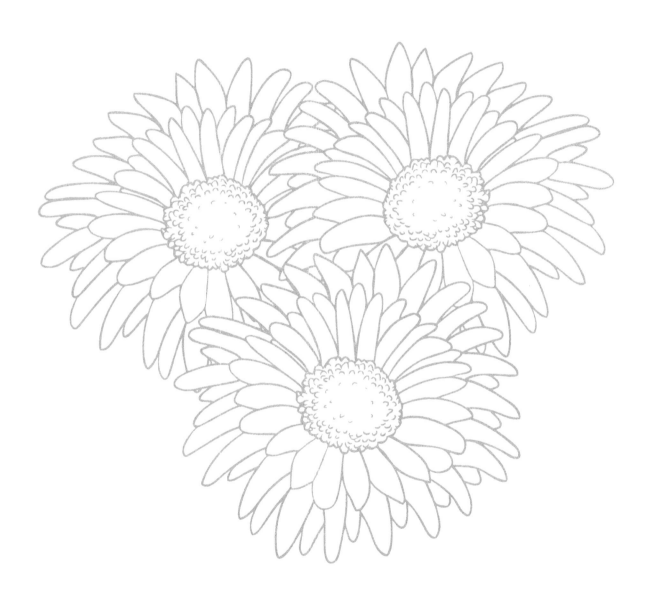

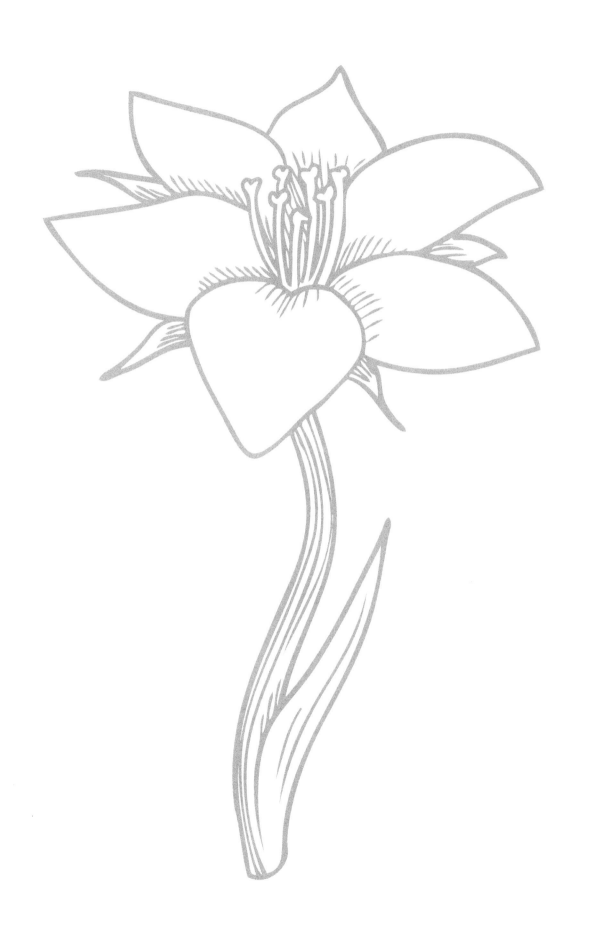

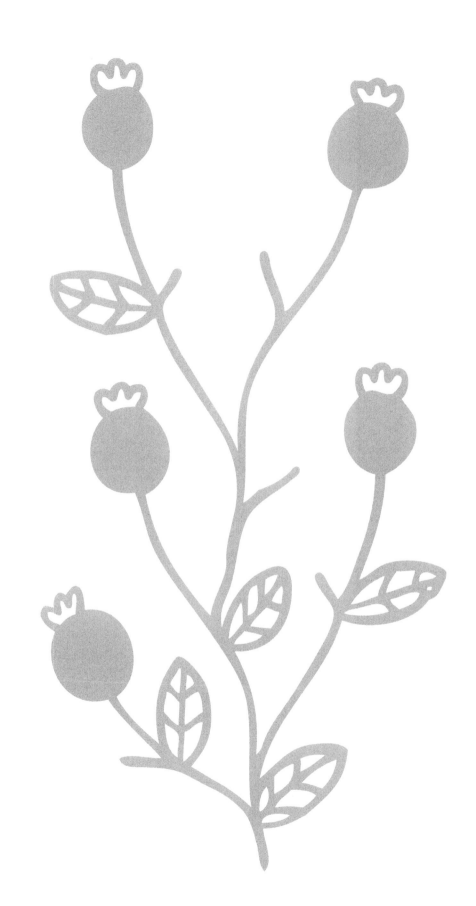

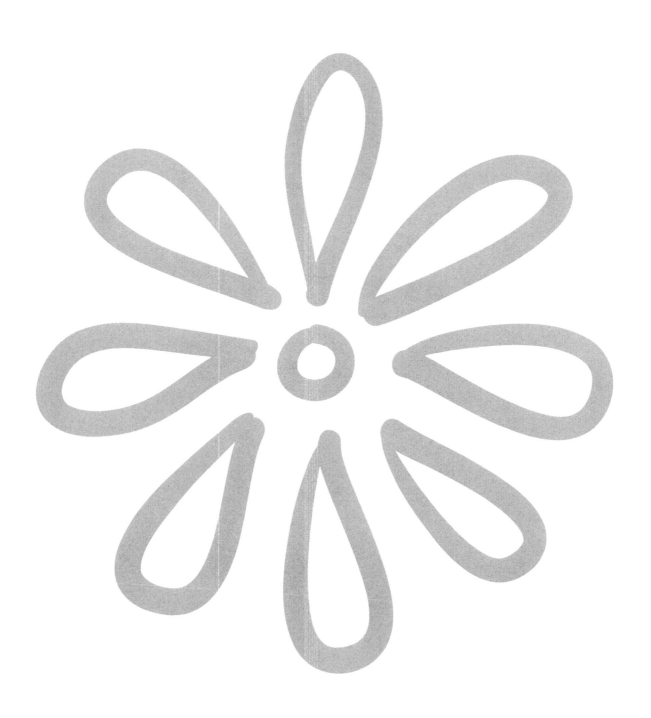

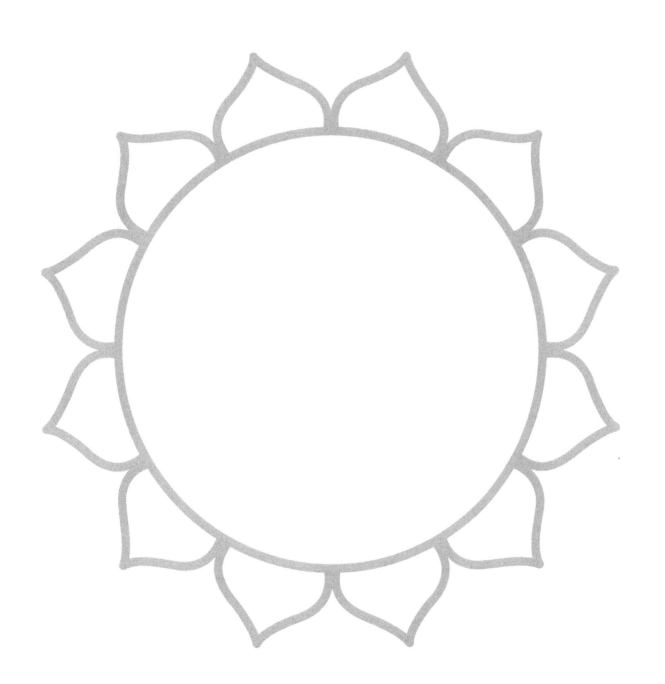

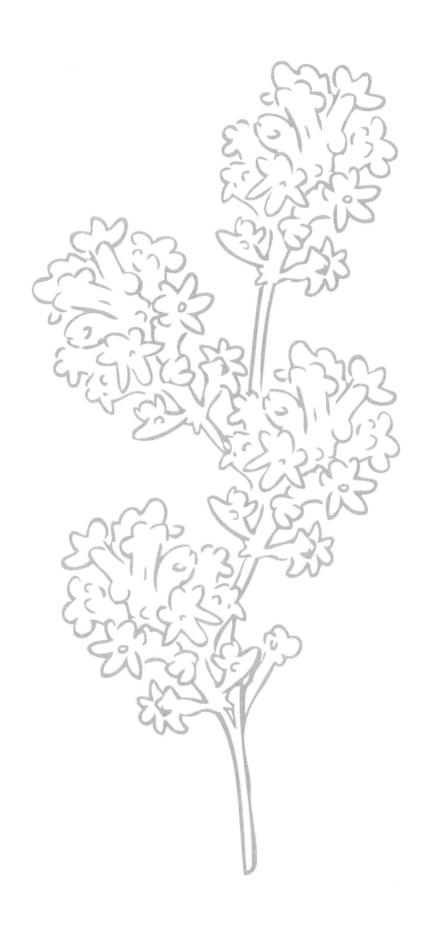

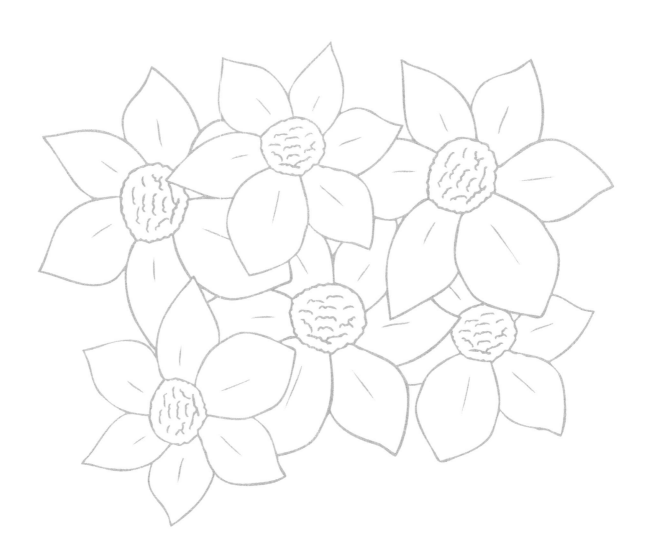

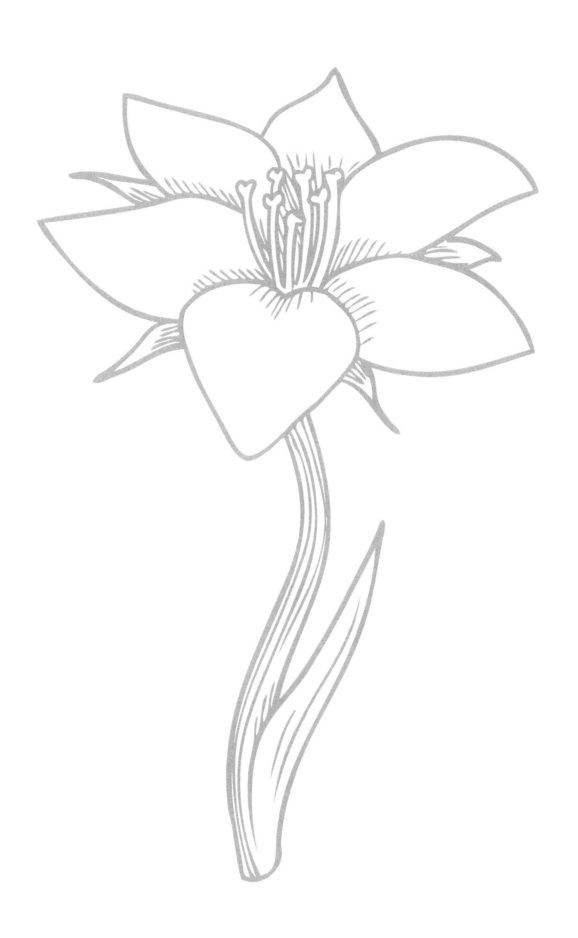

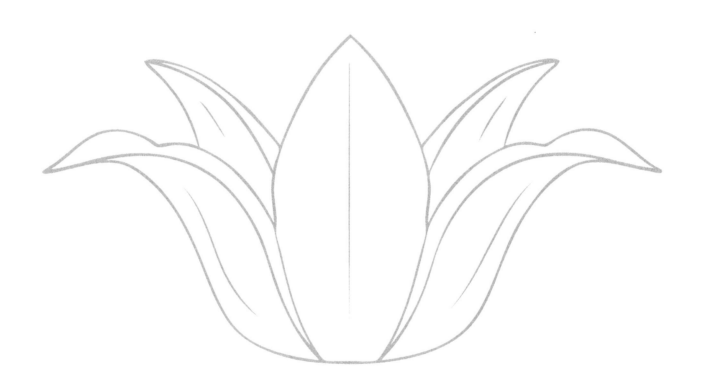

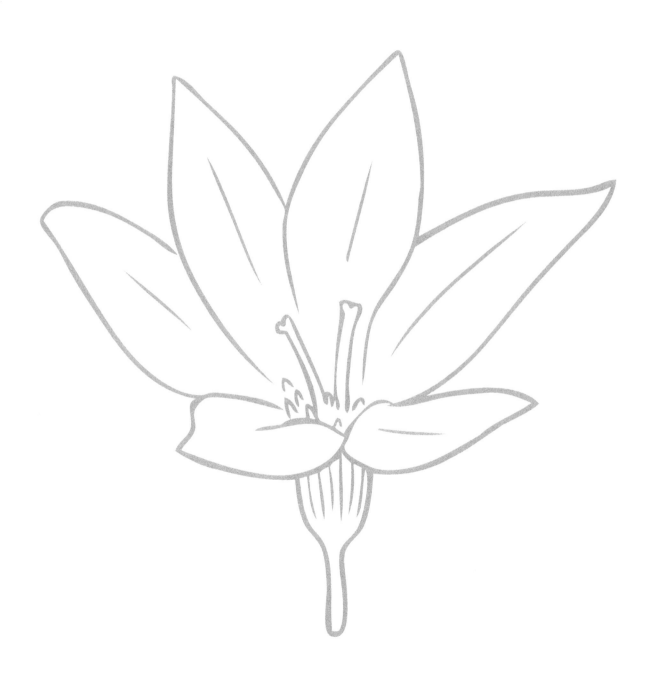

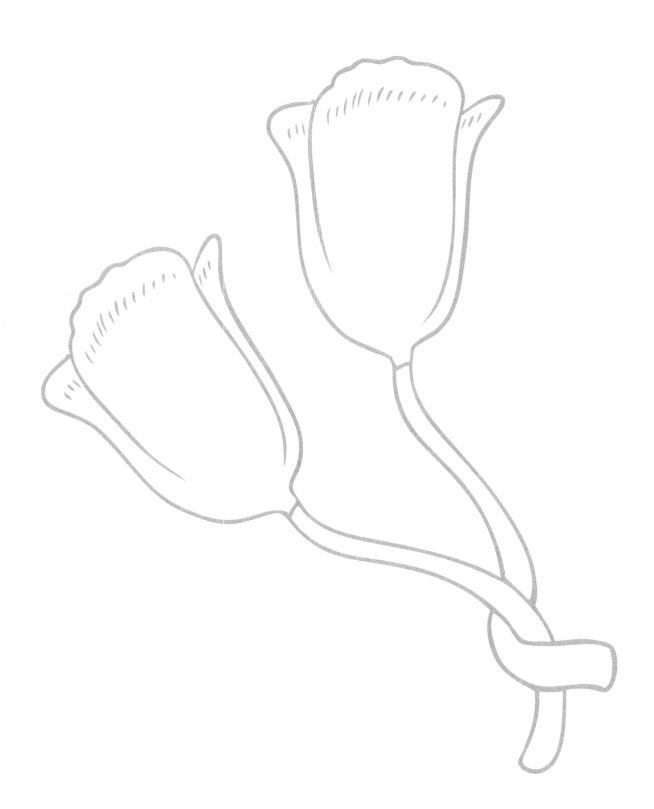

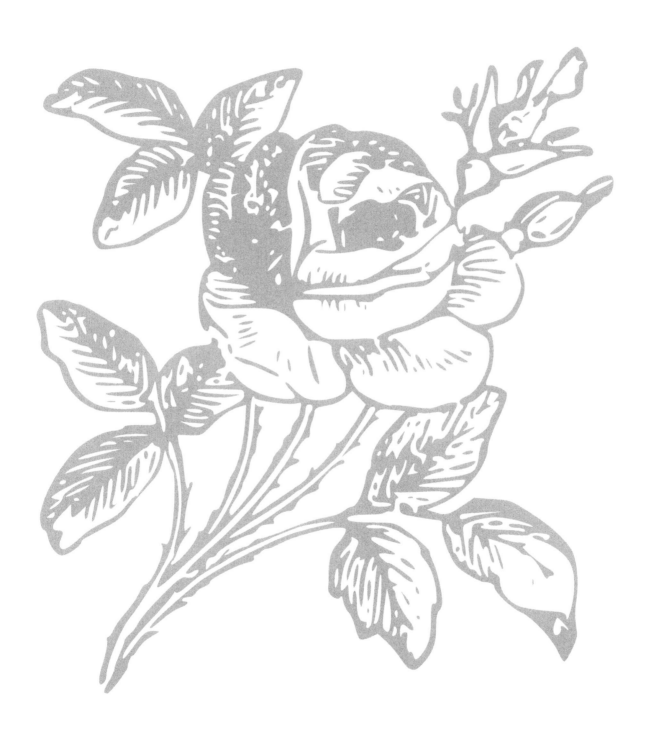

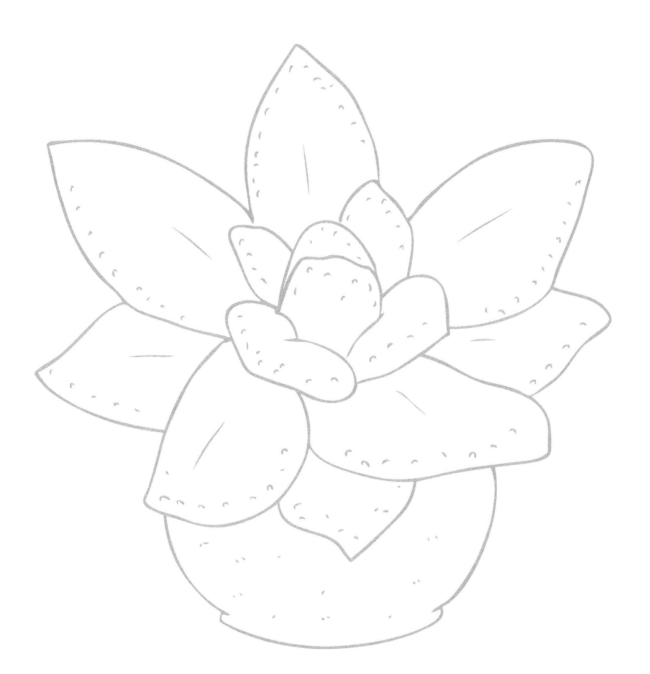

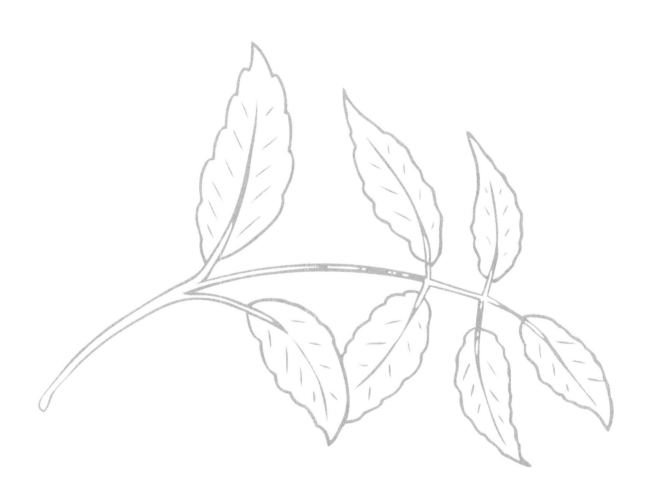

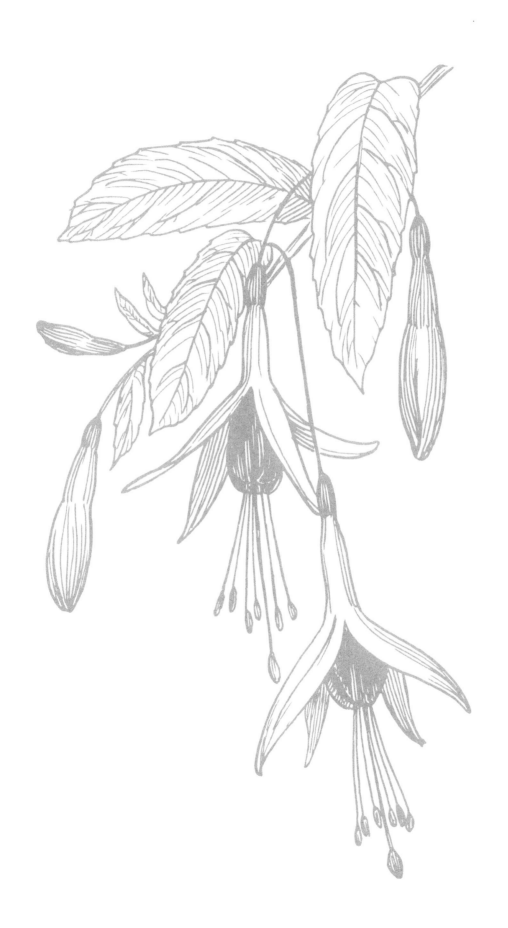

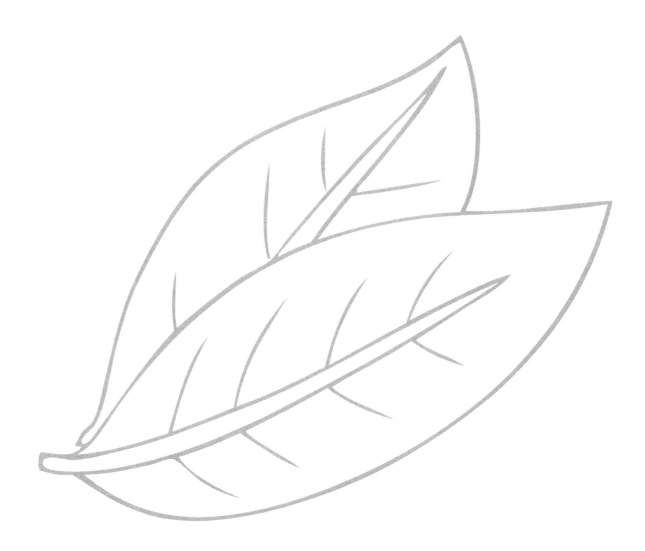

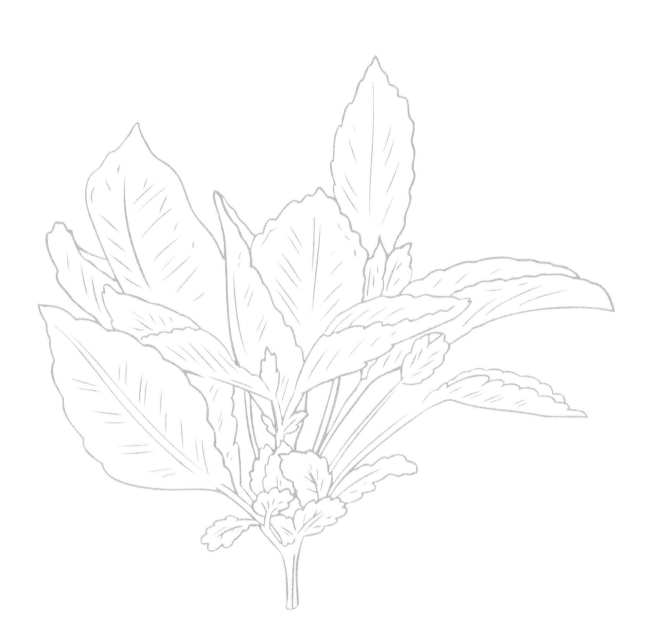

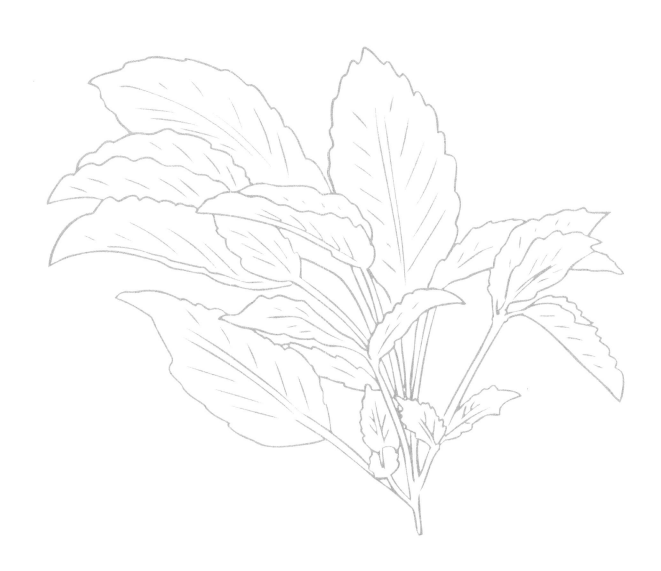

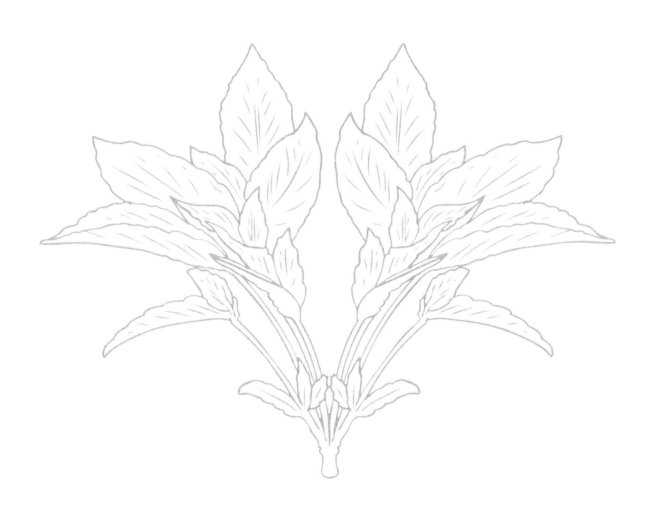

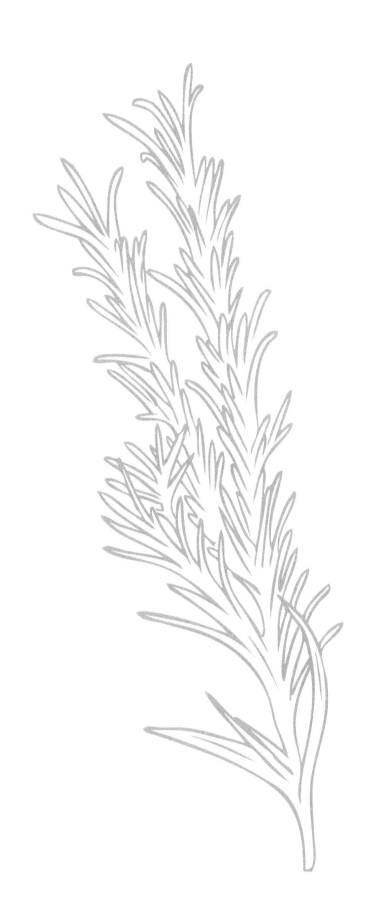

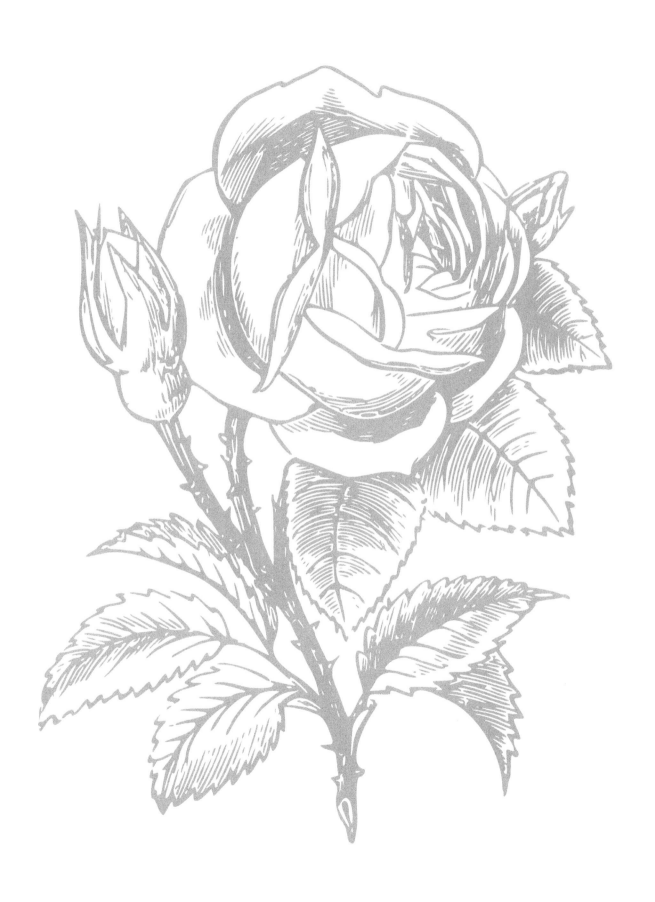

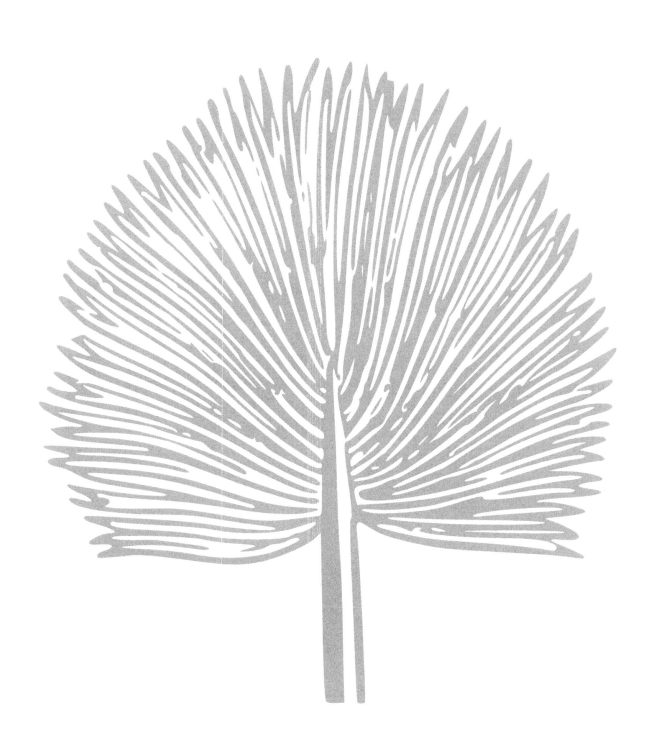

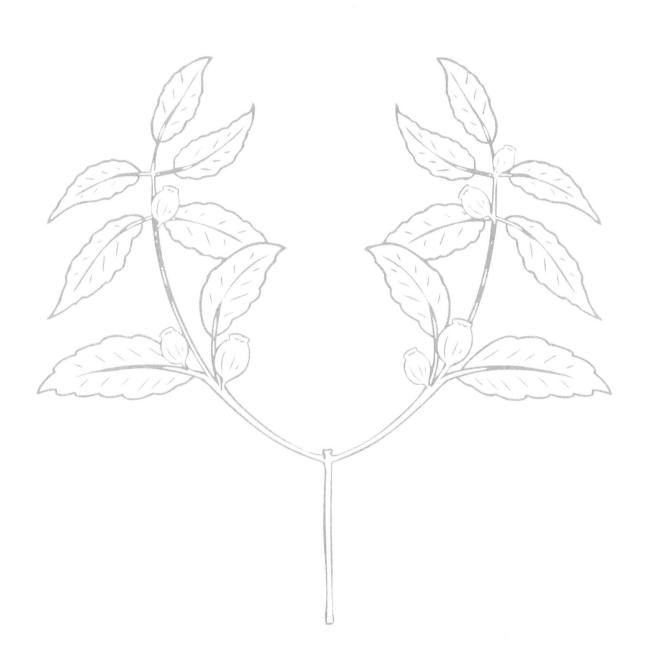

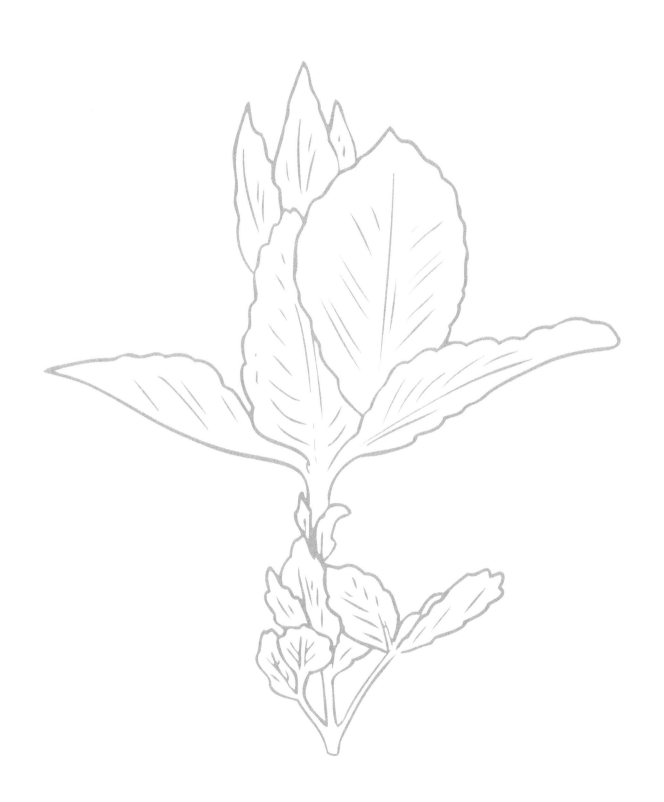

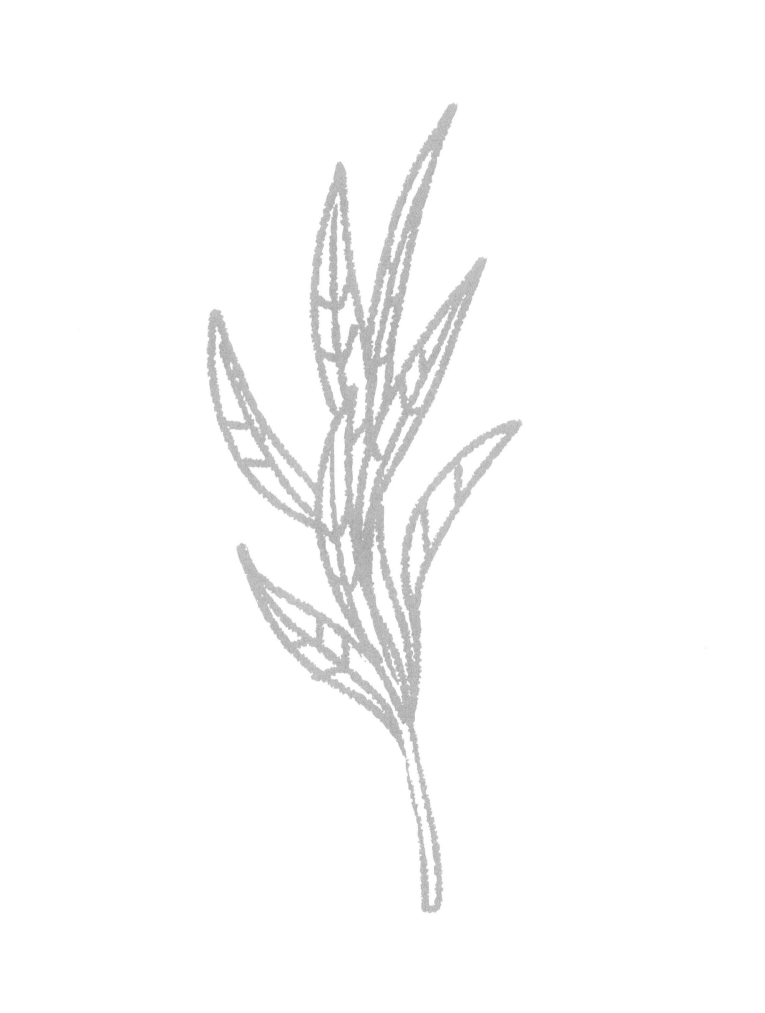

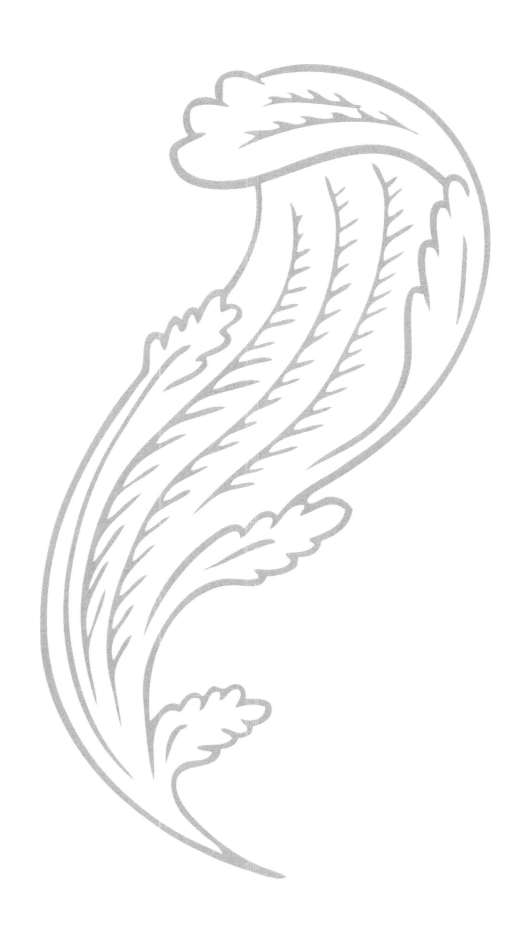

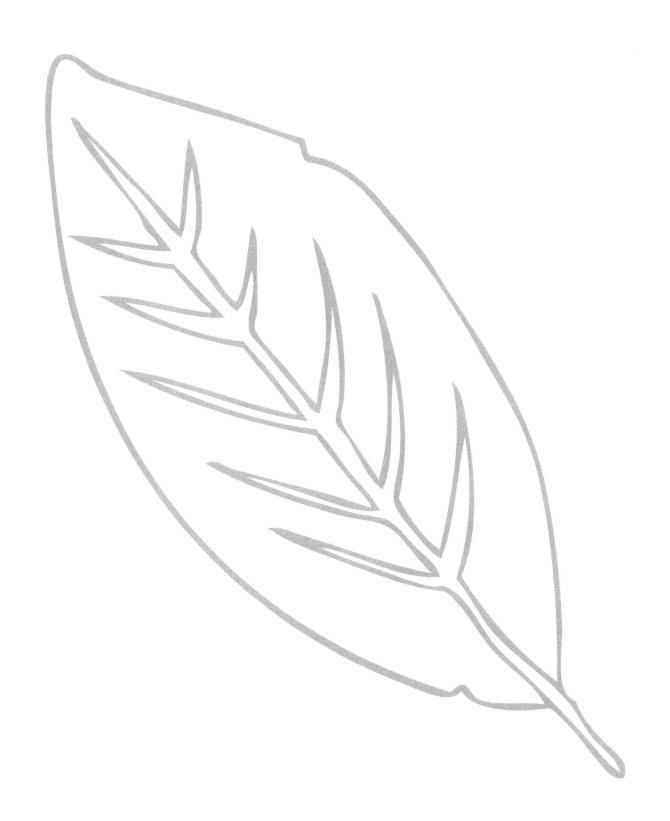

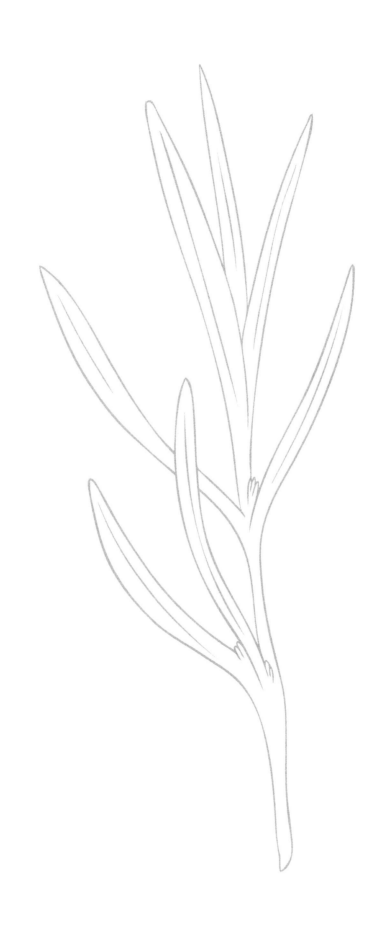

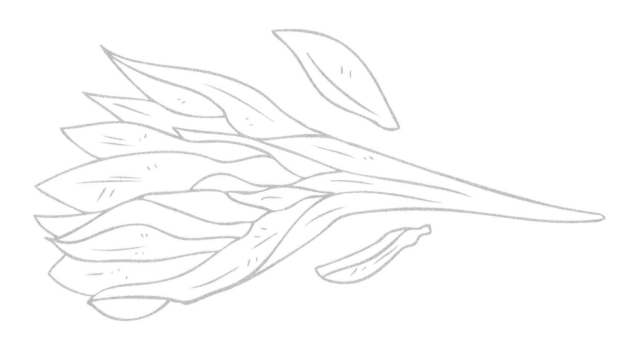

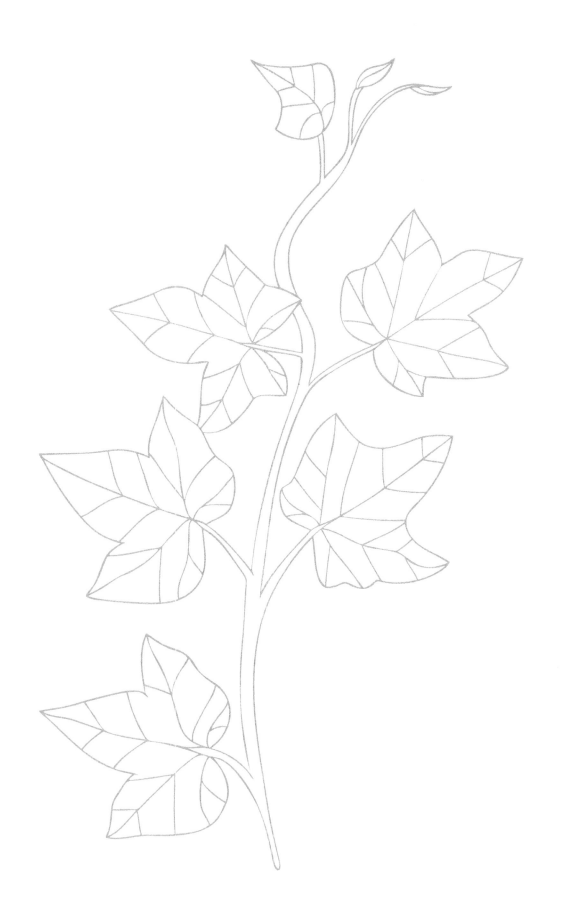

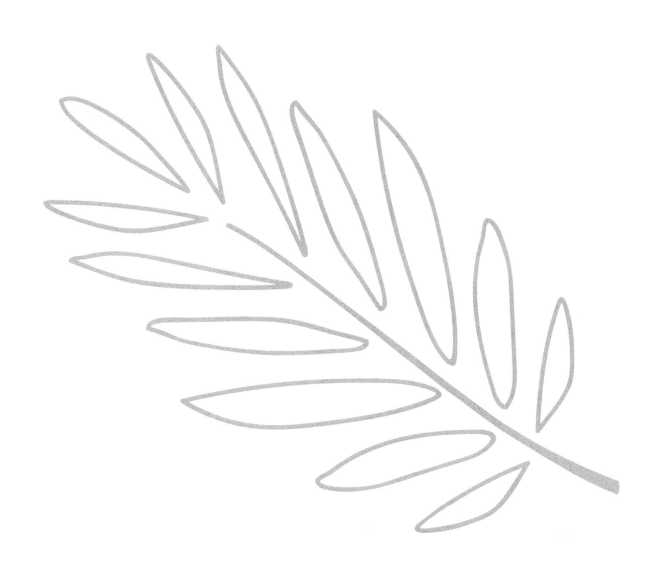

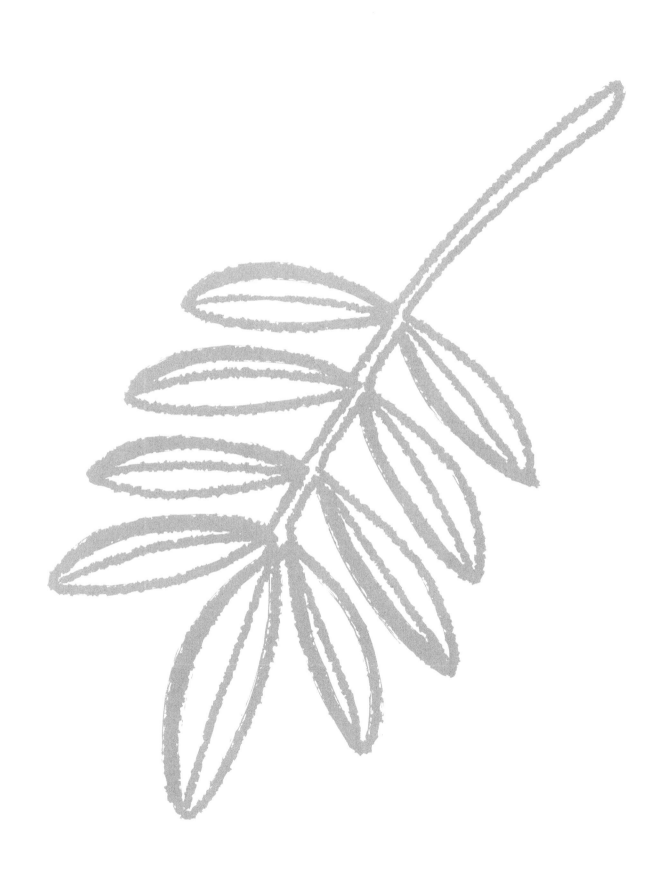

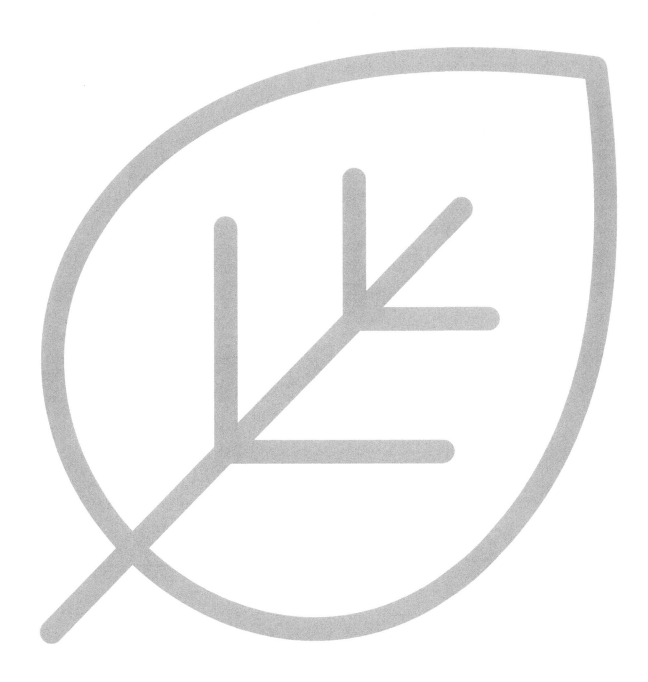

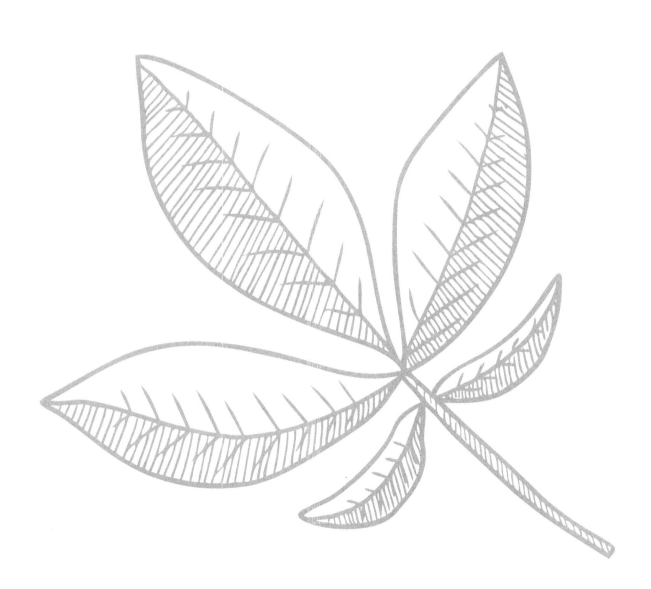

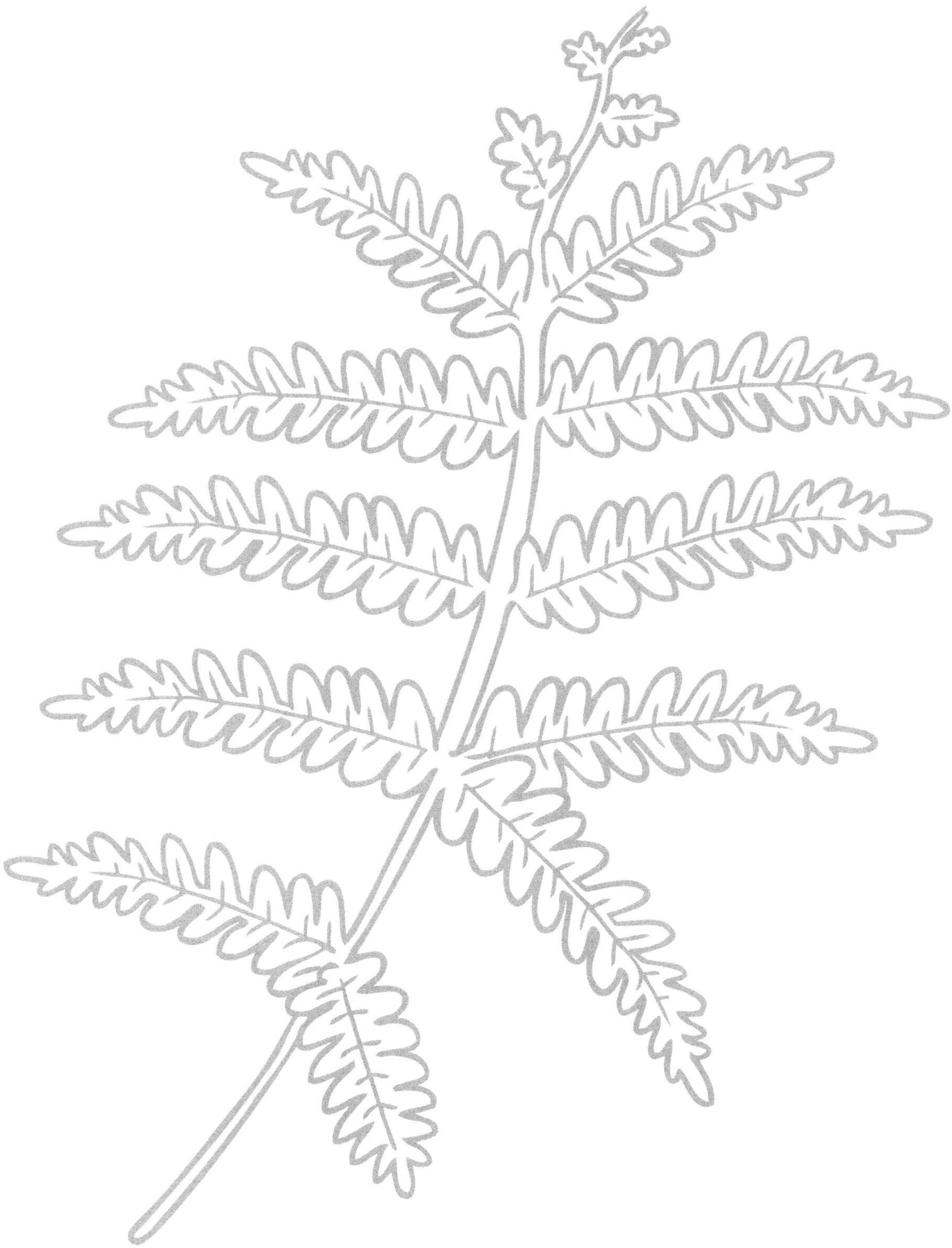

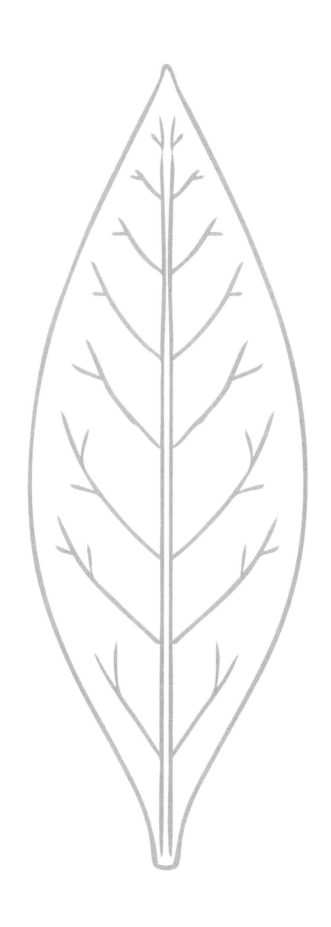

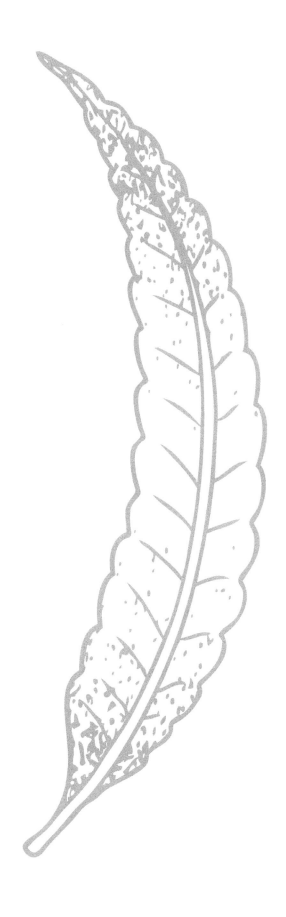

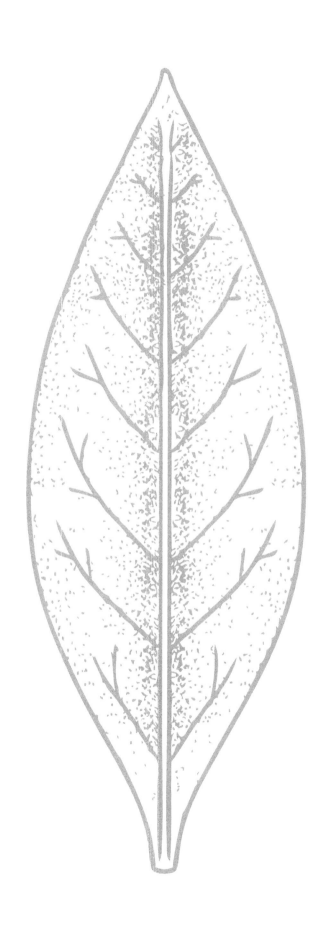

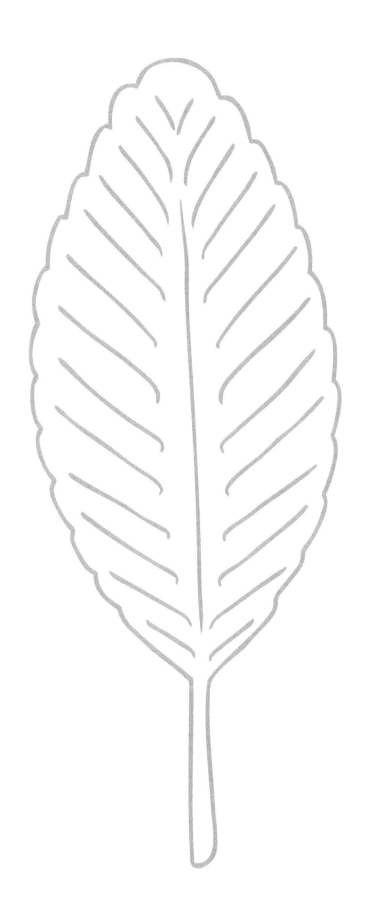

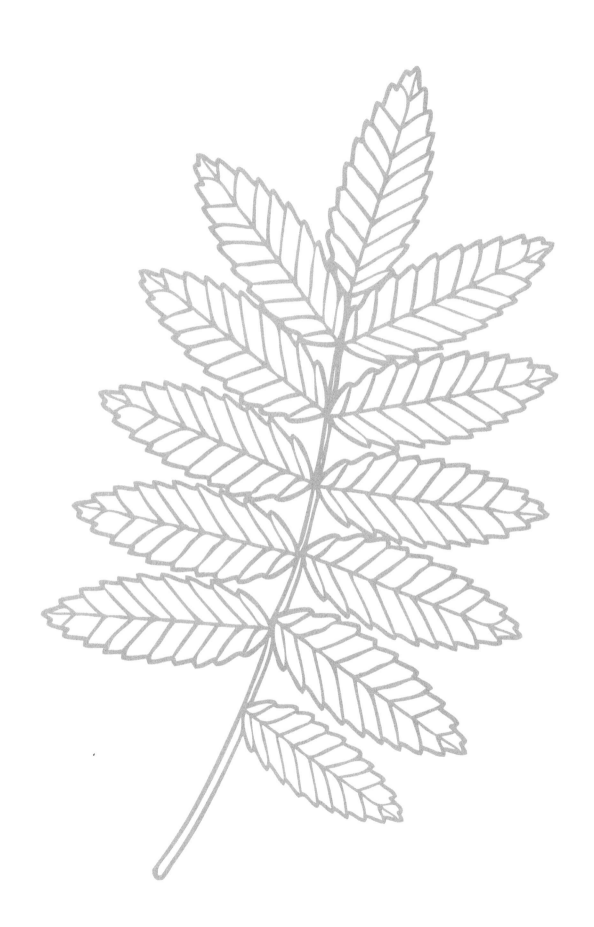

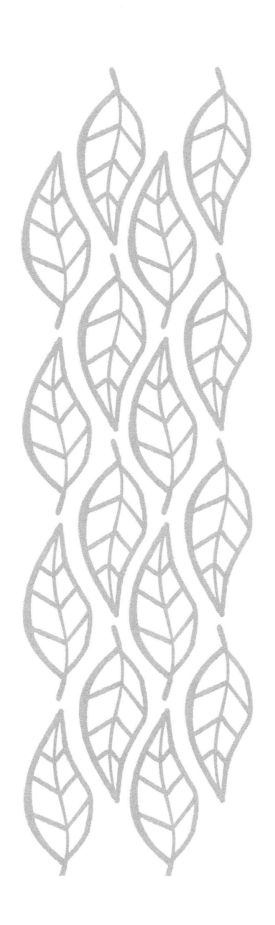

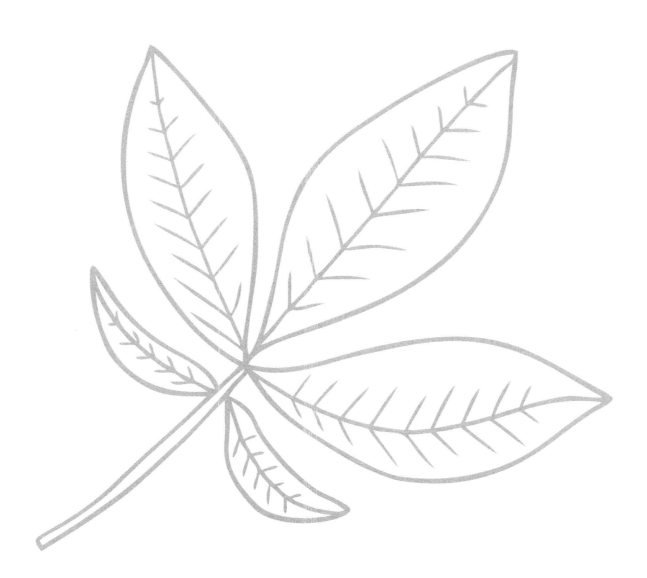

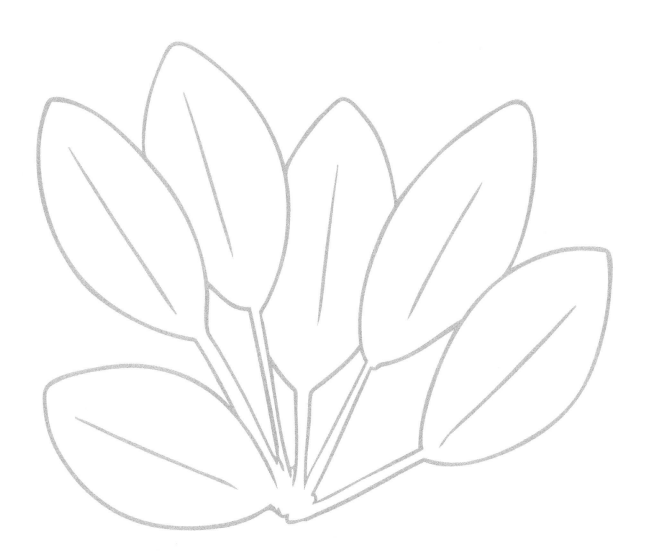

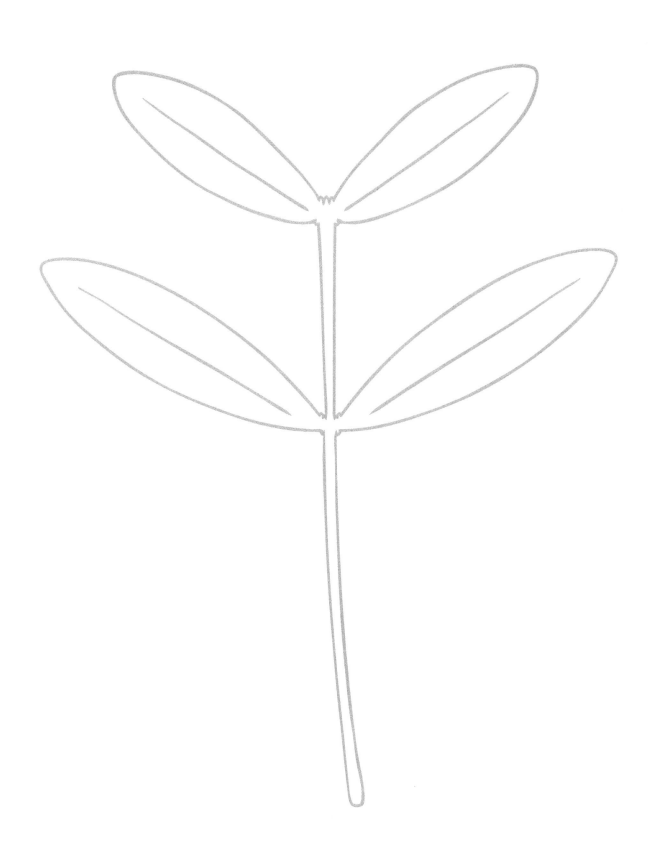

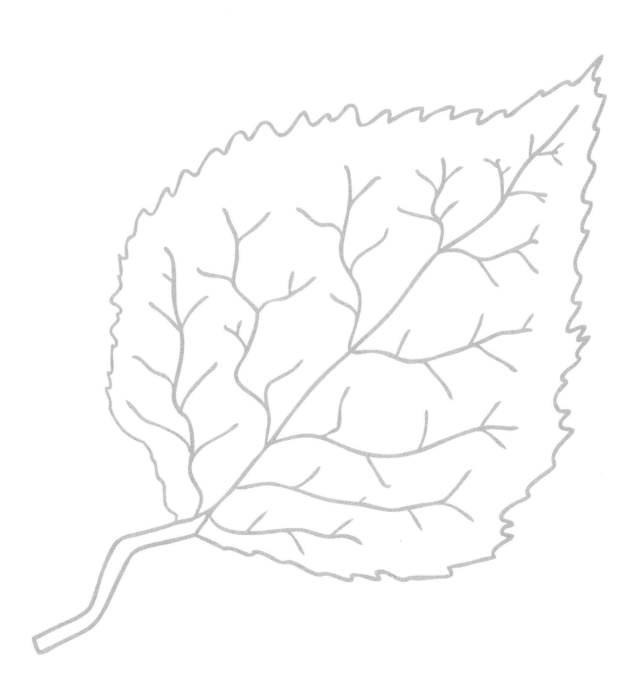

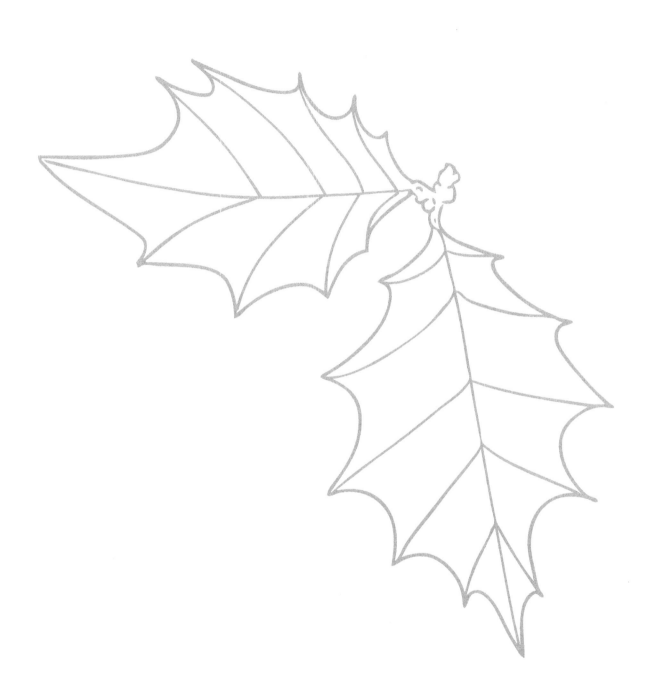